GLUTEN-FREE FOOD LIST

A Comprehensive Guide and Shopping Tips With Food to Eat & Avoid For celiac disease

Patricia D. Stotler

Table of Contents

Introduction

"Are You Tired of Feeling Sick and Confused About What You Can Safely Eat?"

Every day, millions of people struggle with the symptoms of gluten sensitivity and celiac disease, not to mention the confusion and frustration that come with trying to adhere to a gluten-free diet. Do you find yourself asking, "What can I eat that won't make me feel worse?" Imagine a life where you feel vibrant, energetic, and symptom-free. Our book, "Gluten-Free Food List," offers not just a list of foods to eat and avoid, but a gateway to a rejuvenated, healthier you.

Unlock the Benefits of a Gluten-Free Lifestyle

The "Gluten-Free Food List" isn't just a directory; it's a comprehensive guide that transforms your diet and, by extension, your life. Here's how it can capture your attention and benefit you:

1. **Enhanced Health and Well-being**: Learn how eliminating gluten can alleviate symptoms associated with gluten intolerance and celiac disease, such as gastrointestinal distress, inflammation, and fatigue. Feel better daily as your body thanks you for the relief.

2. **Comprehensive Food Lists**: Know exactly what to eat and what to avoid. Our detailed lists include safe gluten-free grains, flours, and hidden sources of gluten in processed foods, helping you make informed choices effortlessly.

3. **Empowering Knowledge**: Understand the nuances of gluten in food labels and restaurant menus, so you can choose wisely and avoid the discomfort that comes with accidental ingestion.

4. **Delicious Recipes and Meal Ideas**: Dive into a collection of tasty, gluten-free recipes that promise to delight your taste buds without compromising your health. From breakfast to dinner, eating gluten-free has never been more enjoyable!

5. **Lifestyle Adaptation Tips**: Learn how to navigate social situations, travel, and dining out without stress. Our guide offers practical advice to maintain your gluten-free lifestyle anywhere, ensuring you stay on track.

6. **Support and Resources**: Gain access to an extensive list of resources, including recommended brands, online tools, and supportive communities that cater to gluten-free individuals.

Managing Objections: What Our Book Offers

We understand that transitioning to a gluten-free diet can be daunting. You might worry about the cost, the availability of food options, or even feel overwhelmed by the need to scrutinize every label. "Gluten-Free Food List" addresses these concerns by offering:

- **Affordable Eating Solutions**: Discover budget-friendly gluten-free foods and tips on how to shop economically without compromising on health.

- **Extensive Availability**: We highlight common and easily accessible gluten-free foods that you can find in any supermarket around you.

- **Simplicity and Clarity**: Our guide breaks down complex nutritional information into easy-to-understand language. Learn how to read labels quickly and identify gluten-free certification marks with ease.

- **Educational Insight**: Build your knowledge about why gluten affects your body the way it does, empowering you with the information needed to advocate for your health.

"Gluten-Free Food List" is more than a book; it's a companion in your journey to a healthier life. Whether you're newly diagnosed with celiac disease, have gluten sensitivity, or simply want to lead a healthier lifestyle, this book is your comprehensive guide to navigating a gluten-free diet with confidence and ease. Join the thousands who have transformed their lives. Start your gluten-free journey today!

Understanding Gluten

Gluten is a protein composite found in wheat and related grains, including barley and rye. It acts as a binder that holds food together and gives dough its elasticity. While it's a vital part of many baking processes, gluten can cause serious health problems for individuals with celiac disease, non-celiac gluten sensitivity, or wheat allergies. When people with celiac disease consume gluten, their immune system mistakenly attacks the small intestine, leading to damage that impedes the absorption of nutrients. This can cause symptoms ranging from gastrointestinal distress, such as bloating and diarrhea, to more severe health issues including nutrient deficiencies, osteoporosis, and increased risk of other autoimmune diseases.

Non-celiac gluten sensitivity, though less severe than celiac disease, also prompts a range of symptoms including stomach pain, fatigue, and headaches when gluten is ingested. This condition does not damage the intestine but can significantly affect quality of life. Those with a wheat allergy, while they react to wheat, do not necessarily react to all forms of gluten, but avoidance of all gluten-containing grains is often recommended to prevent symptoms such as itching, swelling, and in severe cases, anaphylaxis.

Given these risks, maintaining a gluten-free diet is essential for the health and well-being of individuals with these conditions. A gluten-free diet involves eliminating all foods containing or contaminated with gluten. This means avoiding not only obvious sources like breads, pastas, and baked goods but also many processed foods such as soups, sauces, and ready meals which may use gluten as a thickener or stabilizer.

The benefits of following a gluten-free diet for those affected by gluten-related disorders are significant. Symptoms can subside quickly once gluten is removed from the diet, and for those with celiac disease, the intestines often begin to heal, reducing the risk of long-term health complications. Moreover, awareness and understanding of gluten-free dietary needs have increased, making it easier to find suitable and varied alternatives in most food outlets.

People embarking on a gluten-free lifestyle must become vigilant label readers and knowledgeable about the hidden sources of gluten in food products. They must also learn to identify gluten-free grains like rice, quinoa, and corn, which can serve as healthy substitutes in their diet. This vigilance ensures that they can enjoy a diverse and nutritionally balanced diet without the risks posed by gluten ingestion.

Benefits of a Gluten-Free Diet

A gluten-free diet, initially recommended for those with celiac disease, has gained popularity as a beneficial lifestyle choice for a broader audience. By eliminating gluten, a protein composite found in wheat, barley, rye, and their derivatives, individuals often experience relief from gastrointestinal distress, chronic inflammation, and associated fatigue. This dietary adjustment is particularly crucial for people with celiac disease, for whom gluten triggers a harmful immune response that damages the intestine, but it also helps those with non-celiac gluten sensitivity who experience similar, though less severe, symptoms without the autoimmune damage.

Following a gluten-free diet, as detailed in the "Gluten-Free Food List," can lead to improved digestive health, as many report a significant reduction in bloating, gas, diarrhea, and constipation. These changes can occur because the diet helps reduce the chronic inflammation often caused by gluten in sensitive individuals, leading to better overall digestive function. Additionally, the diet's emphasis on whole, unprocessed foods such as fruits, vegetables, meats, and naturally gluten-free grains—like rice and quinoa—contributes to a richer intake of various nutrients.

For individuals with dermatitis herpetiformis, a skin condition associated with celiac disease, a gluten-free diet can lead to a decrease in skin rashes and itching. The diet also benefits those with gluten-related disorders by enhancing their energy levels and reducing the foggy-headed feeling often reported by those with gluten sensitivities.

Furthermore, the structured approach to food selection and increased awareness of food ingredients typically lead to more health-conscious decisions. This informed decision-making can inadvertently lead to weight management benefits. However, it's important to note that gluten-free is not inherently lower in calories; rather, the focus on balanced eating and natural foods helps avoid excessive consumption of processed foods, which are often high in sugars and fats.

Mental health improvements are an often-overlooked benefit of adopting a gluten-free diet. For those sensitive to gluten, removing it can lead to clearer thinking and better emotional health. Some studies suggest that gluten can negatively impact mood and psychological function in sensitive individuals, thus removing it may lead to a noticeable improvement in mood and a decrease in symptoms of depression and anxiety.

The "Gluten-Free Food List" serves as an essential tool in navigating this diet, offering detailed lists of safe foods and those to avoid. This guidance is vital for maintaining a strict gluten-free diet, which is necessary not only to avoid immediate discomfort but also to prevent long-term health complications in those with celiac disease or significant sensitivities.

By adhering to a gluten-free diet and utilizing comprehensive resources like the "Gluten-Free Food List," individuals can experience a substantial improvement in quality of life, encompassing physical health, mental well-being, and overall vitality.

Who Should Follow a Gluten-Free Diet?

People often wonder if a gluten-free diet is right for them. Generally, this diet is essential for individuals with celiac disease, an autoimmune disorder where the ingestion of gluten leads to damage in the small intestine. It is estimated that 1 in 100 people worldwide has this condition, though many remain undiagnosed. Symptoms can range from digestive distress like diarrhea and abdominal pain to non-digestive issues such as anemia, joint pain, and skin rashes, making diagnosis sometimes challenging.

Aside from celiac disease, non-celiac gluten sensitivity (NCGS) is another condition that benefits from a gluten-free diet. Individuals with NCGS experience symptoms similar to those of celiac disease, including foggy mind, depression, abdominal bloating, and diarrhea, but do not test positive for celiac disease. Removing gluten from the diet can lead to significant symptom improvement in these cases.

Furthermore, people with wheat allergies, who experience a traditional allergic reaction to wheat proteins, also find relief when following a gluten-free diet. Though their reaction is to wheat specifically, eliminating all gluten can help avoid cross-contaminations and hidden sources of wheat that might trigger an allergic response.

Additionally, some individuals choose a gluten-free diet for other health-related reasons, including reducing chronic inflammation or managing autoimmune diseases like Hashimoto's thyroiditis. While scientific support for gluten-free diets in the management of conditions other than celiac disease and wheat allergy varies, many report feeling better with the dietary change.

Our "Gluten-Free Food List" book serves as a comprehensive guide for these groups, providing detailed lists of safe foods as well as those to avoid. It also offers practical tips on how to read food labels, manage social situations, and maintain nutritional balance, which is crucial since gluten-free products often lack certain vitamins and minerals found in their gluten-containing counterparts.

This diet is not typically recommended for the general population due to the nutritional challenges and restrictions it presents. For those without gluten-related disorders, there is no proven health benefit to avoiding gluten, and doing so might even lead to dietary deficiencies if not properly managed.

In summary, while a gluten-free diet is medically necessary for some, it is a lifestyle choice for others. Understanding the specific needs and challenges associated with gluten-free eating, as outlined in our book, can help individuals make informed decisions and maintain a balanced, healthy diet while successfully managing their conditions.

Identifying Gluten in Your Diet

Common Sources of Gluten

Gluten is a protein found in several types of grains and is ubiquitous in many food products due to its viscoelastic properties, which provide elasticity and chewiness in baked goods. Recognizing the common sources of gluten is essential for those who need or choose to avoid it.

Wheat is the most prevalent gluten-containing grain and appears in numerous forms. This includes whole wheat, wheat bran, wheat germ, spelt, durum, farro, graham, kamut, semolina, and triticale—a hybrid of wheat and rye. These varieties are staples in bread, pasta, cereals, and many processed foods.

Rye, while used less extensively than wheat, is commonly found in rye bread, rye beer, and some cereals. Barley is another significant source of gluten, used in malt products like malt vinegar, beer, and foods flavored with malt.

Beyond these obvious sources, gluten often lurks in less expected places. Processed foods frequently contain gluten as a thickening agent, stabilizer, or flavor enhancer. This includes salad dressings, sauces, soups, and gravies. Many snack foods, such as pretzels, crackers, and even some chips, also contain gluten.

Soy sauce is a notable example, as it's traditionally brewed with wheat. Other condiments and seasonings, including some ketchups and mustards, might use gluten-containing ingredients. Processed meats such as sausages, hot dogs, and deli meats often include gluten as a binder or filler.

Moreover, beverages can also be hidden sources of gluten. Beer made from barley, malt beverages, and other alcoholic drinks like certain types of vodka and whiskey may contain gluten, although pure distilled spirits are considered gluten-free despite their source.

In the realm of sweets and desserts, gluten is a common component in cakes, pies, cookies, and pastries, all of which typically use wheat flour. It can also appear in ice cream and candy as a thickener or stabilizer.

Our "Gluten-Free Food List" provides detailed insights into these sources, offering alternatives and helping users identify safe products. The book emphasizes the importance of vigilance in checking labels for gluten-containing ingredients, especially derivatives that might not be immediately recognizable. It also educates on gluten-free certifications and labeling laws that make identifying gluten-free products easier and safer for consumers navigating this complex dietary landscape.

By furnishing a thorough understanding of where gluten might hide, the book empowers readers to make informed choices, ensuring they can maintain a strict gluten-free diet effectively and confidently.

Reading Labels for Hidden Gluten

Reading labels to find hidden gluten is a crucial skill for anyone following a gluten-free diet. Gluten, a protein found in wheat, barley, rye, and their derivatives, can appear in many forms and under various names on ingredient lists, making it essential to know what to look for.

Firstly, the obvious ingredients to avoid are wheat, barley, rye, triticale (a cross between wheat and rye), malt (which is usually made from barley), and brewer's yeast. These can appear in foods as flour or thickeners, and in products like beers, malt vinegars, and other malt-based foods.

Beyond these, gluten can hide under less obvious names. For instance, wheat products may be listed as durum, emmer, semolina, spelt, farina, or einkorn. Additionally, many processed foods use ingredients like hydrolyzed vegetable protein, texturized vegetable protein, and natural flavorings, which can be sourced from wheat. Even some medications and vitamins use gluten as a binding agent.

The term "modified food starch" often raises concerns, as this can be made from wheat. Unless it specifically states it's made from a gluten-free source, such as corn, it should be avoided. Similarly, dextrin, a type of starch, can also occasionally be sourced from wheat unless labeled otherwise.

It's also essential to be wary of cross-contamination. Foods labeled as "gluten-free" must meet regulatory standards, which generally require that the food contains less than 20 parts per million of gluten. However, foods processed in facilities that also process wheat or other gluten-containing grains may be subject to cross-contamination unless the manufacturer explicitly states that their production lines are gluten-free.

In the United States, the Food and Drug Administration (FDA) requires that foods labeled "gluten-free," "free of gluten," "no gluten," and "without gluten" must meet the definition of containing less than 20 ppm of gluten. This labeling is voluntary, meaning that not all gluten-free foods will necessarily carry this label, so it's still important to read the ingredient list thoroughly.

Furthermore, some certification organizations offer gluten-free certification for products that meet strict gluten-free standards. These certifications can provide an additional level of assurance beyond the

FDA's requirements, and products that carry these certifications often feature a logo on the packaging.

Finally, to assist in the safe selection of foods, "Gluten-Free Food List" provides comprehensive lists and examples of both safe and unsafe ingredients, helping individuals navigate grocery aisles and menus more confidently. The book emphasizes the importance of continuous vigilance in label reading, as ingredients can change without notice, making it essential to regularly review even familiar products' labels.

Understanding these complexities and staying informed about the various ways gluten can appear in products are vital steps in maintaining a healthy, gluten-free diet.

Gluten-Free Certification and What It Means

Gluten-free certification is a critical tool for individuals following a gluten-free diet, especially for those with celiac disease or gluten sensitivity, as it helps them identify products that are safe to consume. This certification involves a rigorous process where food products, production facilities, and packing processes are inspected for compliance with specific gluten-free standards set by certifying organizations. These standards typically require that foods contain less than 20 parts per million (ppm) of gluten, which is the safe threshold for most people with gluten-related disorders according to international guidelines.

There are several prominent gluten-free certification programs globally, each with its own seal that can be displayed on product packaging. In the United States, for example, the Gluten-Free Certification Organization (GFCO) is one of the most recognized bodies, requiring products to meet strict gluten-free standards that are even more stringent than those required by the FDA for gluten-free labeling. Another significant certification comes from the Celiac Support Association (CSA), which uses a stricter criterion, certifying products that contain less than 5 ppm of gluten.

For consumers, seeing a gluten-free certification seal on a product provides reassurance that the item has been independently verified to meet strict gluten-free standards. This is particularly important because cross-contamination can occur during manufacturing or even through shared facilities, and products without certification may not be safe for those with severe sensitivities or celiac disease.

Certified gluten-free products typically avoid ingredients that are commonly contaminated with gluten, such as oats or natural flavorings, unless those ingredients have also been certified gluten-free. The certification process includes periodic inspections and product testing to ensure continued compliance, providing an additional layer of trust and safety for consumers.

Furthermore, in the "Gluten-Free Food List" book, the importance of these certifications is underscored by providing readers with a guide to understanding different certification seals and what they imply. This guide helps individuals make safer and more informed choices when shopping for gluten-free products. Additionally, the book discusses how to effectively use these certifications in conjunction with reading ingredient labels to avoid gluten exposure, especially considering that not all products labeled "gluten-free" might go through the stringent certification process.

Gluten-free certification is an invaluable asset for those on a gluten-free diet, offering a safeguard against gluten contamination and helping manage a gluten-free lifestyle more effectively. By choosing products that carry a trusted gluten-free certification seal, individuals can significantly reduce the risk of accidental gluten ingestion.

Grains and Cereals

Grain/Cereal	Ingredient	Cooking Instructions	Nutritional Information (per 100g)	Serving Size	Cooking Time
Quinoa	Quinoa seeds	Rinse under cold water. Bring 2 cups water for 1 cup quinoa to a boil, then simmer.	120 kcal, 4g protein, 2g fat, 21g carbs	1 cup cooked	15-20 minutes
Buckwheat	Buckwheat groats	Rinse well. Use 2 cups water for 1	92 kcal, 3.4g protein,	1 cup cooked	10-12 minutes

Grain/Cereal	Ingredient	Cooking Instructions	Nutritional Information (per 100g)	Serving Size	Cooking Time
		cup groats. Bring to a boil, then simmer.	0.62g fat, 19.94g carbs		
Amaranth	Amaranth seeds	Combine 1 cup seeds with 3 cups water. Boil and simmer.	103 kcal, 3.8g protein, 1.6g fat, 18.7g carbs	1 cup cooked	20-25 minutes
Sorghum	Sorghum grains	Use 3 cups water for 1 cup sorghum. Boil and simmer.	96 kcal, 2.7g protein, 0.62g fat, 21g carbs	1 cup cooked	50-55 minutes

Grain/Cereal	Ingredient	Cooking Instructions	Nutritional Information (per 100g)	Serving Size	Cooking Time
Millet	Millet grains	Toast lightly, then add 2 cups water for 1 cup millet. Boil and simmer.	119 kcal, 3.5g protein, 1g fat, 23g carbs	1 cup cooked	25-30 minutes
Teff	Teff grains	Use 3 cups water for 1 cup teff. Bring to a boil, then simmer.	101 kcal, 3.9g protein, 0.65g fat, 19.8g carbs	1 cup cooked	15-20 minutes
Corn (polenta)	Cornmeal	Gradually whisk cornmeal into boiling water. Stir	89 kcal, 1.9g protein, 0.3g fat, 18.7g carbs	1 cup cooked	25-30 minutes

Grain/Cereal	Ingredient	Cooking Instructions	Nutritional Information (per 100g)	Serving Size	Cooking Time
		frequently.			
Rice (brown)	Brown rice	Use 2 ½ cups water for 1 cup rice. Bring to a boil, then simmer.	111 kcal, 2.6g protein, 0.9g fat, 23g carbs	1 cup cooked	45-50 minutes
Rice (white)	White rice	Use 2 cups water for 1 cup rice. Bring to a boil, then simmer.	130 kcal, 2.7g protein, 0.28g fat, 28g carbs	1 cup cooked	18-20 minutes
Wild Rice	Wild rice grains	Use 3 cups water for 1 cup wild	101 kcal, 4g protein, 0.34g fat,	1 cup cooked	45-50 minutes

Grain/Cereal	Ingredient	Cooking Instructions	Nutritional Information (per 100g)	Serving Size	Cooking Time
		rice. Bring to a boil, then simmer.	21.34g carbs		
Oats (certified GF)	GF oats	Use 2 cups water for 1 cup oats. Boil and simmer.	68 kcal, 2.4g protein, 1.4g fat, 12g carbs	1 cup cooked	10-15 minutes
Chia Seeds	Chia seeds	Mix 1 part chia to 6 parts water, let sit until gel forms.	486 kcal, 17g protein, 31g fat, 42g carbs	2 tablespoons raw	No cooking required
Flaxseed	Flaxseed	Ground flaxseed can be added to	534 kcal, 18g protein, 42g fat, 29g	2 tablespoons raw	No cooking required

Grain/Cereal	Ingredient	Cooking Instructions	Nutritional Information (per 100g)	Serving Size	Cooking Time
		smoothies or baked goods.	carbs		
Arrowroot	Arrowroot powder	Mix with a little cold water, then add to hot liquids as a thickener.	357 kcal, 0.3g protein, 0.1g fat, 88g carbs	1 tablespoon	Varied, as thickener
Cassava	Cassava root	Peel, chop, and boil until tender.	160 kcal, 1.36g protein, 0.28g fat, 38.06g carbs	1 cup cooked	20-30 minutes

Proteins

Protein Ingredient	Cooking Instructions	Nutritional Information (per serving)	Serving Size	Cooking Time
Chicken breast	Grill over medium heat until the internal temperature reaches 165°F.	165 calories, 31g protein, 3.6g fat	1 medium breast (approx. 150g)	20-25 minutes
Salmon fillet	Bake at 375°F, seasoned with lemon, dill, and olive oil, until flaky.	233 calories, 25g protein, 15g fat	1 fillet (approx. 140g)	15-20 minutes
Lean ground beef	Pan-fry until fully browned and no pink remains.	218 calories, 26g protein, 13g fat	100g	10-15 minutes
Tofu (firm)	Cube and sauté with soy sauce (gluten-free) and vegetables.	70 calories, 8g protein, 4g fat	100g	10-15 minutes

Protein Ingredient	Cooking Instructions	Nutritional Information (per serving)	Serving Size	Cooking Time
Lentils	Boil in water until tender, can be seasoned as desired.	230 calories, 18g protein, 0.8g fat	1 cup cooked (approx. 200g)	15-20 minutes
Black beans	Rinse and cook in boiling water, season with cumin and garlic.	227 calories, 15g protein, 0.9g fat	1 cup cooked (approx. 172g)	90-120 minutes (if from dry)
Quinoa	Rinse and boil in water or broth until spirals appear.	222 calories, 8g protein, 3.6g fat	1 cup cooked (approx. 185g)	15-20 minutes
Almonds	Raw or roasted, great as a snack or chopped in salads.	164 calories, 6g protein, 14g fat	1 oz (approx. 28g)	N/A
Greek yogurt (plain)	Serve chilled, add fresh fruit or honey for	100 calories, 17g protein, 0.7g fat	1 cup (approx. 245g)	N/A

Protein Ingredient	Cooking Instructions	Nutritional Information (per serving)	Serving Size	Cooking Time
	flavor.			
Cottage cheese	Serve chilled, can be combined with fruits or nuts.	206 calories, 23g protein, 8.5g fat	1 cup (approx. 226g)	N/A
Shrimp	Sauté with garlic and olive oil until pink and opaque.	84 calories, 18g protein, 0.2g fat	100g	5-7 minutes
Turkey breast	Roast in the oven at 325°F until the internal temperature reaches 165°F.	135 calories, 30g protein, 0.7g fat	1 medium slice (approx. 140g)	30-40 minutes per pound
Egg (hard-boiled)	Boil in water for 9-12 minutes, then cool in ice water.	78 calories, 6g protein, 5g fat	1 large egg	9-12 minutes
Pork chop	Grill or broil until the internal	231 calories, 25g protein,	1 chop (approx.	10-15 minutes

Protein Ingredient	Cooking Instructions	Nutritional Information (per serving)	Serving Size	Cooking Time
	temperature reaches 145°F with a 3-minute rest.	13g fat	170g)	
Edamame	Boil or steam pods, sprinkle with sea salt.	189 calories, 17g protein, 8g fat	1 cup shelled (approx. 155g)	5-10 minutes

This table provides a variety of animal-based and plant-based proteins that fit within a gluten-free diet, ensuring ample options for meals throughout the day. Whether you're cooking a quick meal or planning a detailed menu, these protein sources can help maintain a balanced and nutritious gluten-free diet.

Dairy Products

Dairy Product	Ingredients	Instructions	Nutritional Information (per serving)	Serving Size	Cooking/Preparation Time
1. Whole Milk	Milk	Drink as is or use in recipes	150 cal, 8g fat, 12g carbs, 8g protein	1 cup (240 ml)	Ready to use
2. Skim Milk	Fat-free milk	Drink as is or use in recipes	90 cal, 0g fat, 12g carbs, 8g protein	1 cup (240 ml)	Ready to use
3. Yogurt	Milk, live yogurt cultures	Consume alone or mixed with fruits or granola	110 cal, 2.5g fat, 15g carbs, 6g protein	1 cup (245 g)	Ready to use

Dairy Product	Ingredients	Instructions	Nutritional Information (per serving)	Serving Size	Cooking/Preparation Time
4. Greek Yogurt	Milk, cream, live yogurt cultures	Use in smoothies, as a substitute for sour cream, or with honey	100 cal, 4g fat, 6g carbs, 10g protein	1 cup (245 g)	Ready to use
5. Butter	Cream, salt (sometimes)	Use as a spread or in cooking	102 cal, 11.5g fat, 0g carbs, 0.12g protein	1 tablespoon (14 g)	Ready to use
6. Ghee	Butter	Use in place of oils or butter for higher heat	112 cal, 12.7g fat, 0g carbs, 0g protein	1 tablespoon (13 g)	Ready to use

Dairy Product	Ingredients	Instructions	Nutritional Information (per serving)	Serving Size	Cooking/Preparation Time
		cooking			
7. Cheddar Cheese	Milk, salt, enzymes, sometimes annatto	Eat as is, or melt in dishes	113 cal, 9g fat, 0.4g carbs, 7g protein	1 oz (28 g)	Ready to use
8. Mozzarella Cheese	Milk, salt, enzymes	Ideal for topping on pizzas or salads	85 cal, 6g fat, 1g carbs, 6g protein	1 oz (28 g)	Ready to use
9. Cottage Cheese	Milk, cream, salt	Perfect for salads, as a side dish, or in baking recipes	206 cal, 8.2g fat, 6.1g carbs, 23g protein	1 cup (226 g)	Ready to use

Dairy Product	Ingredients	Instructions	Nutritional Information (per serving)	Serving Size	Cooking/Preparation Time
10. Sour Cream	Cultured cream, enzyme	Use as a topping for baked potatoes or in dips	52 cal, 5.1g fat, 1.4g carbs, 0.7g protein	2 tablespoons (30 g)	Ready to use
11. Cream Cheese	Milk, cream, salt, cheese culture, carob	Spread on gluten-free bagels or mix into desserts	99 cal, 9.8g fat, 1.6g carbs, 1.7g protein	1 oz (28 g)	Ready to use
12. Ice Cream	Milk, cream, sugar, flavorings	Serve as a dessert	137 cal, 7g fat, 16g carbs, 2g protein	1/2 cup (65 g)	Ready to serve

Dairy Product	Ingredients	Instructions	Nutritional Information (per serving)	Serving Size	Cooking/Preparation Time
13. Whipping Cream	Cream	Whip for toppings or fold into sauces	52 cal, 5.5g fat, 0.4g carbs, 0.3g protein	1 tablespoon (15 ml)	Ready to use
14. Parmesan Cheese	Milk, salt, rennet	Grate over pasta or salads	110 cal, 7g fat, 1g carbs, 10g protein	1 oz (28 g)	Ready to use
15. Ricotta Cheese	Whey, milk, cream, vinegar	Use in lasagna, stuffed shells, or as a dessert base	180 cal, 14g fat, 3g carbs, 11g protein	1/2 cup (124 g)	Ready to use

Fruit/Vegetable	Ingredient	Nutritional Information (per 100g)	Serving Size	Cooking/Preparation Time
Apple	Fresh apple	Calories: 52, Carbs: 14g, Fiber: 2.4g	1 medium apple	Raw, no cooking required
Banana	Fresh banana	Calories: 89, Carbs: 23g, Fiber: 2.6g	1 medium banana	Raw, no cooking required
Carrot	Fresh carrots	Calories: 41, Carbs: 10g, Fiber: 2.8g	1 medium carrot	Boil/Steam: 10-15 minutes
Spinach	Fresh spinach	Calories: 23, Carbs: 3.6g, Fiber: 2.2g	1 cup	Sauté: 3-5 minutes

Fruit/Vegetable	Ingredient	Nutritional Information (per 100g)	Serving Size	Cooking/Preparation Time
Broccoli	Fresh broccoli	Calories: 34, Carbs: 7g, Fiber: 2.6g	1 cup chopped	Steam: 5-7 minutes
Orange	Fresh orange	Calories: 47, Carbs: 12g, Fiber: 2.4g	1 medium orange	Raw, no cooking required
Kale	Fresh kale	Calories: 49, Carbs: 9g, Fiber: 3.6g	1 cup chopped	Sauté: 5-7 minutes
Strawberry	Fresh strawberries	Calories: 32, Carbs: 8g, Fiber: 2g	1 cup halves	Raw, no cooking required
Sweet Potato	Fresh sweet	Calories: 86, Carbs:	1 medium	Bake: 45 minutes at 400°F

Fruit/Vegetable	Ingredient	Nutritional Information (per 100g)	Serving Size	Cooking/Preparation Time
	potato	20g, Fiber: 3g	potato	
Tomato	Fresh tomato	Calories: 18, Carbs: 4g, Fiber: 1.2g	1 medium tomato	Raw, no cooking required
Blueberry	Fresh blueberries	Calories: 57, Carbs: 14g, Fiber: 2.4g	1 cup	Raw, no cooking required
Zucchini	Fresh zucchini	Calories: 17, Carbs: 3.1g, Fiber: 1g	1 cup sliced	Sauté: 5-7 minutes
Avocado	Fresh avocado	Calories: 160, Carbs: 9g, Fiber: 7g	1 medium avocado	Raw, no cooking required

Fruit/Vegetable	Ingredient	Nutritional Information (per 100g)	Serving Size	Cooking/Preparation Time
Bell Pepper	Fresh bell pepper	Calories: 20, Carbs: 5g, Fiber: 1.7g	1 medium pepper	Raw or Sauté: 5-7 minutes
Cucumber	Fresh cucumber	Calories: 16, Carbs: 3.6g, Fiber: 0.5g	1 medium cucumber	Raw, no cooking required

This table offers a variety of fruits and vegetables that can be incorporated into a gluten-free diet, providing a mix of raw and cooked options that cater to different preferences and nutritional needs. Each entry includes basic instructions for preparation, which can be helpful for those new to cooking or looking to expand their gluten-free diet options. These fruits and vegetables are not only naturally gluten-free but also provide essential nutrients, making them excellent choices for maintaining a balanced diet.

Nuts and Seeds

Ingredient	Description/Instruction	Nutritional Information (per 30g serving)	Serving Size	Cooking Time
Almonds	Raw or roasted without any added gluten-containing ingredients. Great for snacking or added to salads.	170 calories, 6g protein, 15g fat	30g	N/A
Walnuts	Best consumed raw or toasted. Rich in omega-3 fatty acids.	185 calories, 4g protein, 18.5g fat	30g	5-10 mins (toasting)
Cashews	Often found in trail mixes or used to make dairy-free cashew milk and cheese.	165 calories, 5g protein, 13g fat	30g	N/A
Pecans	Usually eaten raw or used in baking. Excellent in pies or candied.	200 calories, 3g protein, 20g fat	30g	N/A

Ingredient	Description/Instruction	Nutritional Information (per 30g serving)	Serving Size	Cooking Time
Brazil Nuts	Consumed raw or blanched. Known for high selenium content.	185 calories, 4g protein, 18g fat	30g	N/A
Pumpkin Seeds	Can be roasted with a dash of salt for a crunchy snack.	158 calories, 7g protein, 13g fat	30g	10-15 mins (roasting)
Sunflower Seeds	Often roasted and salted, used in salads, or as a snack.	174 calories, 6g protein, 15g fat	30g	N/A
Chia Seeds	Used in puddings, smoothies, or as an egg substitute in vegan baking due to their gel-forming capability.	138 calories, 5g protein, 9g fat	30g	N/A
Flaxseeds	Ground flaxseeds are used as an omega-3 boost in smoothies or as a vegan egg substitute.	150 calories, 5g protein, 12g fat	30g	N/A

Ingredient	Description/Instruction	Nutritional Information (per 30g serving)	Serving Size	Cooking Time
Sesame Seeds	Commonly used in baking, on buns, or in Asian cuisine.	160 calories, 5g protein, 14g fat	30g	N/A
Pine Nuts	Often used in pesto or sprinkled over salads for a buttery flavor.	190 calories, 4g protein, 19g fat	30g	N/A
Macadamia Nuts	Known for their high fat content and creamy taste, ideal for cookies and desserts.	204 calories, 2g protein, 21.5g fat	30g	N/A
Hemp Seeds	Added to smoothies, yogurts, or salads for a protein boost.	166 calories, 9.5g protein, 14.6g fat	30g	N/A
Poppy Seeds	Used in baking and on top of bagels.	145 calories, 5g protein, 12g fat	30g	N/A
Pistachios	Eaten on their own as a snack or used to add crunch to salads and	160 calories, 6g protein, 13g fat	30g	N/A

Ingredien t	Description/Instructio n	Nutritional Informatio n (per 30g serving)	Servin g Size	Cookin g Time
	desserts.			

Note: When purchasing nuts and seeds for a gluten-free diet, it's essential to buy those that are labeled as gluten-free to avoid cross-contamination during processing. Some nuts and seeds may be processed in facilities that also handle wheat and other gluten-containing grains, making them unsafe for people with celiac disease or gluten sensitivity.

Fats and Oils

Fats and Oils	Ingredient	Nutritional Information per Serving	Serving Size	Cooking Time	Typical Uses
Olive Oil	100% Olive	120 calories, 14g fat, 0g carbs, 0g protein	1 tbsp	N/A	Dressings, sautéing, drizzling
Coconut Oil	100% Coconut	121 calories, 14g fat, 0g carbs, 0g protein	1 tbsp	N/A	Baking, frying, smoothies
Avocado Oil	100% Avocado	124 calories, 14g fat, 0g carbs, 0g protein	1 tbsp	N/A	High-heat cooking, salads
Canola Oil	100% Canola	124 calories, 14g fat, 0g carbs, 0g protein	1 tbsp	N/A	Frying, baking, marinades

Fats and Oils	Ingredient	Nutritional Information per Serving	Serving Size	Cooking Time	Typical Uses
Flaxseed Oil	100% Flaxseed	120 calories, 14g fat, 0g carbs, 0g protein	1 tbsp	N/A	Cold dishes, supplements
Grapeseed Oil	100% Grapeseed	120 calories, 14g fat, 0g carbs, 0g protein	1 tbsp	N/A	Stir-frying, dressings
Almond Oil	100% Almond	120 calories, 14g fat, 0g carbs, 0g protein	1 tbsp	N/A	Salad dressings, desserts
Walnut Oil	100% Walnut	120 calories, 14g fat, 0g carbs, 0g protein	1 tbsp	N/A	Finishing oil for dishes, dressings
Sesame Oil	100% Sesame	120 calories, 14g fat, 0g carbs, 0g	1 tbsp	N/A	Asian cooking, flavoring

Fats and Oils	Ingredient	Nutritional Information per Serving	Serving Size	Cooking Time	Typical Uses
		protein			
Macadamia Nut Oil	100% Macadamia	120 calories, 14g fat, 0g carbs, 0g protein	1 tbsp	N/A	Baking, salad dressings
Peanut Oil	100% Peanut	119 calories, 14g fat, 0g carbs, 0g protein	1 tbsp	N/A	Deep frying, stir-frying
Sunflower Oil	100% Sunflower	120 calories, 14g fat, 0g carbs, 0g protein	1 tbsp	N/A	General cooking, salad dressings
Clarified Butter (Ghee)	100% Butter	112 calories, 13g fat, 0g carbs, 0g protein	1 tbsp	N/A	Indian cooking, baking

Fats and Oils	Ingredient	Nutritional Information per Serving	Serving Size	Cooking Time	Typical Uses
Lard	100% Pork Fat	115 calories, 13g fat, 0g carbs, 0g protein	1 tbsp	N/A	Baking, frying
Palm Oil	100% Palm	120 calories, 14g fat, 0g carbs, 0g protein	1 tbsp	N/A	Baking, frying, flavoring

This table serves as a useful reference for individuals following a gluten-free diet, providing a variety of fat and oil options that are not only safe but also beneficial for diverse cooking methods and culinary applications. Each listed fat and oil is inherently gluten-free, ensuring they are suitable for gluten-sensitive diets. Always ensure to purchase these oils in their pure, unblended forms to avoid any potential cross-contamination with gluten-containing substances.

Snacks and Convenience Foods

Snack/Convenience Food	Ingredients	Instructions	Nutritional Information (per serving)	Serving Size	Cooking/Preparation Time
1. Almond Flour Crackers	Almond flour, sea salt, egg	Mix ingredients, roll out dough, cut into shapes, and bake.	160 calories, 6g protein, 14g fat	10 crackers	15 min prep, 12 min bake
2. Rice Cakes	Whole grain brown rice, salt	Compress rice and steam.	35 calories, 0.7g protein, 0.3g fat, 7.3g	1 cake	Ready to eat

Snack/Convenience Food	Ingredients	Instructions	Nutritional Information (per serving)	Serving Size	Cooking/Preparation Time
			carbs		
3. Veggie Chips	Sweet potatoes, beets, carrots, olive oil, salt	Slice veggies, toss with oil and salt, bake until crispy.	150 calories, 2g protein, 9g fat, 16g carbs	1 cup	10 min prep, 20 min bake
4. Gluten-Free Pretzels	Gluten-free flour blend, yeast, sugar, salt,	Create dough, shape into pretzels, boil, and bake.	100 calories, 3g protein, 0.5g fat, 22g carbs	30g	1 hr prep, 20 min bake

Snack/Convenience Food	Ingredients	Instructions	Nutritional Information (per serving)	Serving Size	Cooking/Preparation Time
	baking soda				
5. Hummus Dip	Chickpeas, tahini, lemon juice, garlic, olive oil	Blend ingredients until smooth.	70 calories, 2g protein, 5g fat, 4g carbs	2 tablespoons	10 min prep
6. Gluten-Free Granola	Oats (gluten-free), honey, almonds, dried fruit	Mix ingredients, spread on tray, bake until	200 calories, 6g protein, 8g fat, 28g carbs	1/2 cup	10 min prep, 30 min bake

Snack/Convenience Food	Ingredients	Instructions	Nutritional Information (per serving)	Serving Size	Cooking/Preparation Time
		golden.			
7. Fruit Leather	Pureed fruit (choice), honey, lemon juice	Spread pureed fruit on baking sheet, bake at low heat.	45 calories, 0.5g protein, 0g fat, 10g carbs	1 strip	5 min prep, 3-4 hrs bake
8. Popcorn	Popcorn kernels, olive oil, salt	Pop kernels in oil, season with salt.	106 calories, 3g protein, 6g fat, 12g	3 cups	5 min prep, 3 min cook

Snack/Convenience Food	Ingredients	Instructions	Nutritional Information (per serving)	Serving Size	Cooking/Preparation Time
			carbs		
9. Roasted Chickpeas	Chickpeas, olive oil, paprika, garlic powder, salt	Toss chickpeas with oil and spices, bake until crispy.	120 calories, 5g protein, 4g fat, 18g carbs	1/2 cup	10 min prep, 40 min bake
10. Cheese Sticks	Cheese (such as cheddar or mozzarella)	Cut cheese into sticks.	80 calories, 5g protein, 6g fat, 1g carbs	1 stick	Ready to eat

Snack/Convenience Food	Ingredients	Instructions	Nutritional Information (per serving)	Serving Size	Cooking/Preparation Time
11. Nut Mix	Mixed nuts (almonds, walnuts, pecans), sea salt	Mix nuts and salt.	200 calories, 5g protein, 18g fat, 5g carbs	1/4 cup	Ready to eat
12. Gluten-Free Muffins	Gluten-free flour blend, eggs, sugar, blueberries, milk	Mix ingredients, pour into muffin tins, and bake.	150 calories, 3g protein, 4g fat, 25g carbs	1 muffin	15 min prep, 25 min bake
13. Yogurt Parfait	Greek yogurt, gluten-	Layer yogurt, granola,	220 calories, 12g	1 cup	5 min prep

Snack/Convenience Food	Ingredients	Instructions	Nutritional Information (per serving)	Serving Size	Cooking/Preparation Time
	free granola, fresh berries	and berries in a cup.	protein, 3g fat, 34g carbs		
14. Banana Chips	Bananas, lemon juice, cinnamon	Slice bananas, toss with lemon juice and cinnamon, bake.	100 calories, 1g protein, 0g fat, 26g carbs	1 cup	10 min prep, 2 hrs bake
15. Energy Balls	Dates, oats (gluten-free), peanut	Blend ingredients, roll into balls,	100 calories, 3g protein, 5g fat,	1 ball	15 min prep, 1 hr chill

Snack/Convenience Food	Ingredients	Instructions	Nutritional Information (per serving)	Serving Size	Cooking/Preparation Time
	butter, flax seeds	chill.	12g carbs		

Foods to Avoid on a Gluten-Free Diet

Grains Containing Gluten

For individuals following a gluten-free diet, particularly those with celiac disease or gluten sensitivity, avoiding certain grains is crucial to manage health and prevent symptoms. Gluten is a protein found in various grains, and it can cause health issues for those with gluten-related disorders.

Grain	Contains Gluten Because	Why to Avoid
1. Wheat	Contains gliadin, a gluten protein that triggers adverse autoimmune responses in those with celiac disease.	Can cause digestive harm, nutrient malabsorption, and severe health complications in sensitive individuals.
2. Barley	Has hordein, a form of gluten, which can cause similar reactions as wheat gluten.	Leads to inflammation and digestive issues in gluten-intolerant people.

Grain	Contains Gluten Because	Why to Avoid
3. Rye	Contains secalin, a gluten protein, known to be problematic for those with gluten-related disorders.	Triggers symptoms such as abdominal pain, diarrhea, and even neurological effects in affected individuals.
4. Spelt	Although an ancient wheat variety, it contains gluten similar to modern wheat.	Causes the same negative health effects as wheat, making it unsuitable for those on a gluten-free diet.
5. Kamut	A type of wheat known to contain gluten.	Can provoke symptoms of celiac disease or gluten sensitivity due to its gluten content.
6. Triticale	A hybrid of wheat and rye, thus naturally containing gluten.	Combines the gluten-containing properties of both wheat and rye, increasing the risk of adverse reactions.
7. Farro (Emmer)	An ancient wheat species that contains gluten.	Although often marketed as a health food, its gluten content can cause reactions

Grain	Contains Gluten Because	Why to Avoid
		in sensitive individuals.
8. Bulgur	Made from cracked wheat, thus inherently containing gluten.	Often used in salads and side dishes but should be avoided by those with gluten intolerance.
9. Durum	A type of hard wheat used to make pasta and contains gluten.	Although high in protein, its gluten content can cause gastrointestinal distress in sensitive individuals.
10. Einkorn	An ancient wheat variety that naturally contains gluten.	Even though it's considered less hybridized, it still poses a risk for those with celiac disease.
11. Couscous	Made from semolina flour derived from durum wheat, containing gluten.	Can cause symptoms of gluten intolerance such as cramping, bloating, and fatigue.

Grain	Contains Gluten Because	Why to Avoid
12. Seitan	Made directly from wheat gluten and often used as a meat substitute in vegetarian diets.	It is pure gluten, making it one of the most dangerous foods for those with gluten-related disorders.
13. Matzo	Traditionally made from wheat flour and water.	As it contains wheat, it is unsuitable for those on a gluten-free diet during Passover or any other time.
14. Beer (from barley)	Most beers are brewed from barley, a gluten-containing grain.	Regular beer must be avoided as it contains gluten unless specifically labeled gluten-free.
15. Malt (from barley)	Derived from barley and used in various products, including cereals and snacks.	Contains gluten that can lead to gastrointestinal issues and other symptoms in those with gluten sensitivities.

Avoiding these grains is crucial for maintaining a strict gluten-free diet, which is the only effective treatment for managing celiac disease and mitigating symptoms of gluten sensitivity. Substituting these grains with gluten-free alternatives like rice, corn, quinoa, and certified gluten-free oats can help maintain dietary variety and nutritional balance. This approach ensures that those affected by gluten-related disorders can enjoy a healthy, diverse diet without experiencing adverse health effects.

Processed Foods Commonly Containing Gluten

For individuals on a gluten-free diet, avoiding processed foods that commonly contain gluten is crucial. Gluten, a protein found in wheat, barley, rye, and triticale, can cause serious health complications for those with celiac disease, non-celiac gluten sensitivity, or wheat allergy. Below is a table that lists 15 processed foods commonly containing gluten and explains why they should be avoided.

Processed Food	Common Sources of Gluten	Reason to Avoid
1. Bread and Pastries	Wheat flour, barley malt	Wheat flour is a primary ingredient in most commercial breads, making them high in gluten.
2. Pasta	Wheat	Traditional pastas are made from wheat and contain gluten, which can trigger symptoms in sensitive individuals.

Processed Food	Common Sources of Gluten	Reason to Avoid
3. Cereals	Wheat, barley, malt flavoring	Many breakfast cereals include gluten-containing ingredients or are processed in facilities with gluten cross-contact.
4. Biscuits and Crackers	Wheat flour, barley malt extract	These often contain wheat as a main ingredient and are at high risk for containing gluten.
5. Processed Meats	Fillers made from wheat, barley malt flavoring	Gluten is often used as a binder or filler in products like sausages, hot dogs, and deli meats.
6. Soups and Sauces	Wheat flour as a thickener, barley	Many canned or boxed soups and sauces use wheat flour as a thickening agent, hidden source of gluten.
7. Beer and Malt Beverages	Barley, malt	Most beers and malt beverages are brewed from

Processed Food	Common Sources of Gluten	Reason to Avoid
		barley, which contains gluten.
8. Snack Foods (e.g., pretzels)	Wheat flour	Snack foods, including pretzels and some chips, are typically made with wheat flour.
9. Salad Dressings and Condiments	Wheat flour, malt vinegar	Gluten may be used as a thickener or flavor enhancer in dressings and condiments.
10. Flavored Coffees and Teas	Barley, flavor additives	Some flavored coffees and teas include barley-based additives or other gluten-containing ingredients.
11. Imitation Meats	Wheat gluten (seitan)	Imitation or mock meats often use seitan, which is made from wheat gluten, as a primary protein source.
12. Desserts	Cookies, cake	Gluten is often present in

Processed Food	Common Sources of Gluten	Reason to Avoid
and Ice Cream	pieces, and other mix-ins that contain wheat	mix-ins or flavor bases in many processed desserts and ice creams.
13. Candy and Chocolate	Barley malt, wheat flour, modified food starch	Certain candies and chocolates might contain gluten as fillers or flavor enhancers.
14. Instant and Flavored Rice	Seasoning mixes containing wheat or barley	Seasoning packets often contain hidden gluten, which can contaminate otherwise gluten-free rice.
15. Gravies and Seasoning Mixes	Wheat flour	Commonly used as thickening agents in these products, wheat flour is a major source of gluten.

Hidden Sources of Gluten

Hidden Source of Gluten	Commonly Found In	Reason to Avoid
1. Soy Sauce	Sauces, marinades, and some Asian dishes	Often made with wheat; can trigger gluten-related symptoms. Gluten-free alternatives are available.
2. Imitation Crab	Sushi, seafood salads	Typically made from fish paste and wheat to mimic the texture of crab.
3. Licorice	Candy	Usually contains wheat flour as a binder.
4. Bouillon Cubes	Soups, broths, and stews	Often have wheat as a stabilizer or flavor enhancer.
5. Salad Dressings	Bottled dressings and mixes	May contain wheat-based thickeners or malt vinegar derived from barley.
6. Seitan	Vegan and vegetarian meat substitutes	Made entirely from gluten (wheat protein) to mimic meat texture.

Hidden Source of Gluten	Commonly Found In	Reason to Avoid
7. Modified Food Starch	Processed foods, condiments, and medications	Often sourced from wheat, although it can come from other sources; labeling is key to identification.
8. Malt	Cereals, snacks, and beverages	Derived from barley and contains gluten.
9. Communion Wafers	Religious services	Typically made from wheat. Gluten-free alternatives should be requested if necessary.
10. Beer and Malt Beverages	Alcoholic beverages	Made from barley malt. Gluten-free beers are made specifically without gluten-containing grains.
11. Meatballs and Meatloaf	Packaged or restaurant-prepared dishes	Often use breadcrumbs as a binder. Gluten-free versions should use gluten-free bread.
12. Soups and Broths	Canned or boxed varieties	May use wheat flour as a thickener. Home-made or specifically labeled gluten-

Hidden Source of Gluten	Commonly Found In	Reason to Avoid
		free products are safer choices.
13. Medications and Vitamins	Prescription and over-the-counter drugs	Some pills use gluten as a binding agent. Always check with the manufacturer if not labeled gluten-free.
14. Blue Cheeses	Cheeses	Some are made using bread mold, which could introduce gluten. Check for gluten-free labeling.
15. Gravies and Sauces	Thickened sauces or gravy mixes	Commonly thickened with flour. Look for cornstarch or another gluten-free thickener as an alternative.

Planning Your Gluten-Free Diet

Setting Up Your Gluten-Free Kitchen

Setting up a gluten-free kitchen is essential for those diagnosed with celiac disease, gluten sensitivity, or for anyone adopting a gluten-free lifestyle. It involves more than just stocking up on gluten-free products; it requires a thoughtful approach to avoid cross-contamination and ensure that every meal is safe to consume.

The first step in establishing a gluten-free kitchen is to purge it of all gluten-containing items. This includes obvious sources like breads, pastas, and cereals made from wheat, barley, and rye, but also less obvious sources such as condiments, sauces, and bulk-bin items that may have come into contact with gluten. Once these items are removed, thorough cleaning of the kitchen is necessary. This means washing all cookware, utensils, dishes, and surfaces to remove any gluten residues.

Replacing certain kitchen essentials with gluten-free versions is crucial. This includes purchasing a separate toaster for gluten-free breads, as well as separate cutting boards, colanders, and cooking utensils that will only be used for gluten-free cooking and preparation. Some might even choose to have separate sections or cabinets for storing gluten-free products to avoid any mix-ups.

When shopping for new kitchen supplies, it's important to read labels meticulously. Look for products that are certified gluten-free. These products have undergone testing and are verified to contain less than 20 parts per million (ppm) of gluten, which is safe for most people with gluten sensitivities.

In addition to careful selection of food and kitchenware, the way food is stored and prepared should be adjusted. Always use clean oil for frying and do not use the same oil that was used to cook gluten-containing foods. Similarly, when grilling, either thoroughly clean the grill before use or cook gluten-free foods on aluminum foil to prevent contact with residues of gluten-containing foods.

Awareness and education are key elements of maintaining a gluten-free kitchen. Everyone in the household should be aware of the importance of preventing gluten cross-contamination. This includes understanding the need to use clean utensils, not using the same butter or condiment jars used on gluten-containing bread, and always wiping down surfaces before preparing gluten-free meals.

Finally, creating a supportive kitchen environment involves continuous learning and adapting. Subscribing to gluten-free cooking blogs, joining online communities, and keeping updated with the latest gluten-free products can help in making informed choices and keeping the gluten-free kitchen well-stocked with safe and delicious options. By maintaining strict kitchen protocols and staying informed, individuals and families can enjoy a diverse and enjoyable gluten-free diet safely and easily.

Shopping Tips for Gluten-Free Products

Shopping for gluten-free products requires a level of diligence and knowledge to ensure that the foods chosen are truly free from gluten and safe for individuals with celiac disease, gluten sensitivity, or those choosing a gluten-free diet for other health-related reasons. Here are several practical tips to aid in the selection of gluten-free products:

Firstly, always read labels carefully. In the United States, the FDA requires that gluten-free products contain less than 20 parts per million of gluten. Labels will often indicate whether a product is gluten-free, but it's important to also check for phrases like "made in a facility that also processes wheat," which may suggest a risk of cross-contamination.

Secondly, look for certification seals from reputable organizations such as the Gluten-Free Certification Organization (GFCO), which certifies products that meet strict gluten-free standards. These certifications provide an extra layer of assurance beyond the basic labeling requirements.

Shopping in stores with dedicated gluten-free sections can make the process easier and safer, as these products are less likely to have been cross-contaminated with gluten-containing foods. However, even products in gluten-free sections should be checked for labels and certifications as standards can vary.

Understanding the common sources of hidden gluten helps avoid products that might unexpectedly contain gluten. Foods like soups, sauces, and processed meats can often have gluten-containing ingredients, so always check the ingredient list for things like wheat flour, barley, rye, malt, brewer's yeast, and oats that are not labeled gluten-free.

Becoming familiar with brands that specialize in gluten-free products can also simplify shopping. Many brands offer a wide range of products, from bread and pasta to snacks and desserts, and are generally reliable in maintaining gluten-free standards.

When in doubt, opt for whole, unprocessed foods. Fresh fruits, vegetables, meats, and most dairy products are naturally gluten-free. These can be safer choices and also contribute to a healthier overall diet.

Technology can also be an ally in shopping for gluten-free products. Numerous apps are available that can scan barcodes and provide information on whether a product is gluten-free and safe for your specific dietary needs.

Lastly, when shopping online, use trusted websites that offer a wide variety of gluten-free products. Online shopping can provide access to a broader selection of gluten-free foods and makes it easier to access customer reviews that can attest to the quality and safety of the products.

By employing these strategies, individuals can more effectively navigate the complexities of shopping for gluten-free products, ensuring they maintain a safe and healthy diet.

Gluten-Free Meal Planning and Recipes

Meal planning on a gluten-free diet requires careful consideration to ensure all meals are balanced, satisfying, and, most importantly, gluten-free. This involves selecting a variety of foods that meet nutritional needs without containing gluten, which can be a challenge for those newly diagnosed with celiac disease or gluten sensitivity.

One effective strategy for gluten-free meal planning is to focus on naturally gluten-free foods such as fruits, vegetables, meats, fish, dairy, and gluten-free grains like rice, quinoa, and buckwheat. Planning meals around these items minimizes the risk of gluten exposure and ensures a variety of nutrients are included in the diet.

For breakfast, a simple and nutritious option could be a smoothie made with Greek yogurt, a banana, mixed berries, and a spoonful of gluten-free oatmeal for extra fiber. Another choice might be scrambled eggs with sautéed vegetables and a side of gluten-free toast topped with avocado.

Lunches could be composed of hearty salads with mixed greens, cherry tomatoes, cucumbers, grilled chicken, and a sprinkle of nuts, dressed with a gluten-free vinaigrette. Alternatively, a gluten-free wrap filled with hummus, sprouts, carrots, sliced bell peppers, and turkey slices makes a filling meal.

Dinners can vary from stir-fries using gluten-free tamari sauce instead of soy sauce, served over rice, to more elaborate dishes like gluten-free pasta with a homemade marinara sauce and meatballs made with gluten-free breadcrumbs. Fish or chicken baked with herbs and served with steamed vegetables or a quinoa salad can also provide a satisfying evening meal.

Snacks are essential in a gluten-free diet to maintain energy levels throughout the day. Options include mixed nuts, yogurt with fruit, popcorn made with olive oil and a dash of salt, or carrot sticks with almond butter.

When it comes to baking or desserts, using gluten-free flour blends can allow for the creation of favorite treats like cookies, muffins, or pancakes. It's important to experiment with different flours to find the best blend for each recipe. Almond flour, for instance, adds a rich, nutty flavor to baked goods and is excellent for making gluten-free breads and pastries.

To simplify the meal planning process, it's beneficial to create a weekly menu and shopping list that highlights gluten-free products and ingredients. This not only saves time but also reduces the risk of accidental gluten ingestion. Batch cooking and freezing meals in portions is another helpful strategy, ensuring that there are always gluten-free options readily available.

Additionally, incorporating international cuisines such as Mexican, Japanese, or Indian, which traditionally include many naturally gluten-free dishes, can add variety and excitement to the diet. Dishes like sushi (with gluten-free tamari), corn tortilla tacos, or Indian curries using gluten-free spices are delicious and easy to prepare.

By focusing on naturally gluten-free foods, reading labels carefully, and planning ahead, maintaining a gluten-free diet through thoughtful meal planning and diverse recipes can be both enjoyable and health-promoting. The "Gluten-Free Food List" book provides an extensive collection of recipes and tips that make this easier, helping to ensure that those on a gluten-free diet can eat well and feel great every day.

Living Gluten-Free: Tips and Tricks

Dining Out on a Gluten-Free Diet

Dining out on a gluten-free diet can be a challenging experience, but with proper planning and communication, it can also be a rewarding one. The key to successful dining is preparation and clear communication with the restaurant staff about your dietary needs.

Before choosing a restaurant, it's beneficial to do some research. Many restaurants now offer gluten-free menus or menu items that are marked as gluten-free. Checking the restaurant's website or calling ahead can provide insights into whether they can accommodate gluten-free diets and how seriously they take cross-contamination issues. Apps and websites dedicated to reviewing gluten-free dining experiences can also be helpful.

When at the restaurant, communicating your needs clearly and effectively to the server is crucial. It's important to specify that you are on a gluten-free diet due to health reasons and not just as a dietary preference. This can make the staff take your request more seriously. Ask specific questions about how the food is prepared and whether there is a risk of cross-contamination with gluten-containing foods. For example, inquire if the fries are fried in the same oil used for breaded items, or if the same grill is used for both gluten-free and gluten-containing products.

Bringing a dining card that lists your dietary restrictions can be helpful. These cards can be handed to the chef or the manager to ensure the cooking staff is fully aware of your needs. Dining cards are especially useful in ethnic restaurants where language barriers might make it difficult to communicate your dietary restrictions.

Choose simpler dishes as they are less likely to contain hidden sources of gluten. Grilled meats, salads (without croutons), and steamed vegetables are often safe choices. However, always double-check on marinades, dressings, and sauces, as these can be hidden sources of gluten.

Be aware of cross-contamination in the kitchen. Even if a dish is prepared gluten-free, using the same utensils, cookware, or even toasters for gluten-containing and gluten-free foods can lead to cross-contamination. It's important to ask about these practices and ensure that the kitchen uses separate equipment or thoroughly cleans equipment before preparing your meal.

If possible, dine during less busy hours when the kitchen staff can pay more attention to your specific needs. This also gives you an opportunity to discuss your dietary restrictions without feeling rushed.

Finally, always express gratitude to the server and kitchen staff for accommodating your needs. Positive reinforcement can make the dining experience more pleasant for both parties and encourages the restaurant to continue taking dietary restrictions seriously.

By taking these steps, dining out on a gluten-free diet can be a less daunting task. With the right preparation and communication, you can enjoy a variety of dining experiences while still adhering to your gluten-free requirements.

Handling Social Situations and Gatherings

Navigating social situations and gatherings while maintaining a gluten-free diet requires preparation, communication, and sometimes, a bit of creativity. For many, these events can be a source of stress, especially when the focus is on food, which is often the case. One effective strategy is to plan ahead by contacting the host in advance. This not only ensures that there will be safe food options available but also reduces the anxiety that can come with uncertainty. Explaining one's dietary restrictions to a host can be done in a respectful and non-demanding way, emphasizing health needs rather than personal preference.

Bringing one's own food to gatherings is another practical solution. This could be a gluten-free dish to share, ensuring there's something safe to eat while also introducing others to gluten-free options. This approach can serve as a conversation starter, educating others about gluten-free diets and potentially reducing future dining complications with the same group.

At restaurants or catered events, choosing safe options is easier when one has familiarity with which foods are typically gluten-free and understanding how food is prepared. Calling the restaurant ahead or speaking with the chef upon arrival can provide the necessary assurance that the meal will be safe to consume. Many restaurants are now accustomed to accommodating special dietary requirements and may offer gluten-free menus or meal modifications.

Understanding cross-contamination is also vital. At buffets or potlucks, using clean serving utensils and plates, and serving oneself before gluten-containing dishes are passed around can minimize the risk. It's helpful to be first in line or to ask for portions to be set aside beforehand.

In social settings, there's often pressure to partake in whatever is being offered, but maintaining a gluten-free diet requires assertiveness and, occasionally, the need to politely decline food that might be unsafe. Practicing how to decline offers gracefully, with simple explanations, can ease these interactions. It can be beneficial to focus on the company rather than the food, redirecting conversation to shared interests and experiences beyond eating.

Lastly, support from friends and family can significantly ease the burden. Educating close companions about the implications of gluten exposure can turn them into advocates who can assist in communication and food preparation for social gatherings.

By using these strategies, individuals following a gluten-free diet can manage social situations with confidence, ensuring their health needs are met while still enjoying the company of others.

Traveling While Gluten-Free

Traveling while adhering to a gluten-free diet can present unique challenges, but with the right preparation and strategies, it can be both enjoyable and safe. Before embarking on a trip, thorough research is essential. This involves looking up gluten-free restaurant options at the destination, checking if local cuisine has common gluten-free dishes, and identifying nearby grocery stores that offer gluten-free products.

Packing is also a critical aspect of travel for someone with gluten intolerance or celiac disease. Bringing along gluten-free snacks and staples is advisable, as these can serve as a reliable food source when gluten-free options are scarce. Items such as gluten-free crackers, trail mix, and bars are convenient. Additionally, packing essential cooking supplies like a small cutting board, a travel toaster, and disposable utensils can minimize the risk of cross-contamination.

When flying, travelers should contact the airline in advance to request a gluten-free meal. Since not all airlines can accommodate this, having gluten-free snacks on hand is a good backup plan. For road trips, planning the route with stops that include locations known for accommodating gluten-free diets can make the journey more comfortable.

Upon arrival, communicating dietary needs is paramount, especially when dining out. Learning key phrases in the local language or using a gluten-free restaurant card that explains the dietary restrictions in the local language can significantly aid this process. Additionally, digital resources like gluten-free restaurant finder apps and websites can be invaluable tools for finding suitable dining options.

Accommodation selection can also enhance a gluten-free travel experience. Booking a room with a kitchenette, or at least a refrigerator and microwave, allows for greater control over food preparation and storage. This is particularly useful for longer stays.

Joining local gluten-free groups on social media platforms can provide insights and recommendations on gluten-free dining and shopping options. These groups often share the most up-to-date information, which can be more specific than general tourist guides.

Lastly, it's important to be prepared for the possibility of accidental gluten exposure. Traveling with information on local pharmacies and carrying gluten-digestion aids recommended by a healthcare provider can help manage symptoms should they arise.

By planning ahead, carrying necessary supplies, and utilizing technology, individuals can maintain their gluten-free diet while experiencing the joys of travel. This proactive approach not only ensures dietary safety but also enhances the overall travel experience, allowing travelers to explore new cultures and cuisines without the stress of dietary restrictions.

Health and Nutrition on a Gluten-Free Diet

Nutritional Considerations and Supplements

Maintaining a balanced and nutritious diet is essential for individuals following a gluten-free lifestyle, as it can be challenging to obtain all necessary nutrients while avoiding gluten-containing foods. Here are some nutritional considerations and supplement recommendations to ensure optimal health on a gluten-free diet:

1. Fiber Intake: Many gluten-containing grains are significant sources of dietary fiber. When eliminating these grains, it's essential to find alternative sources of fiber to support digestive health. Incorporating gluten-free grains like quinoa, brown rice, and buckwheat, as well as ample fruits, vegetables, nuts, and seeds, can help maintain adequate fiber intake.

2. Vitamin and Mineral Deficiencies: Gluten-free diets may be deficient in essential nutrients such as iron, calcium, vitamin D, and B vitamins. To address these deficiencies, focus on incorporating nutrient-rich, naturally gluten-free foods into your diet. Additionally, consider supplementation under the guidance of a healthcare professional to ensure you meet your nutritional needs.

3. Calcium: Since many gluten-containing products are also significant sources of calcium, individuals on a gluten-free diet may need to pay extra attention to their calcium intake. Incorporate dairy products, fortified plant-based milk alternatives, leafy greens, and calcium-fortified foods to maintain bone health.

4. Vitamin D: Vitamin D deficiency is common among individuals with celiac disease. While sunlight exposure is an excellent source of vitamin D, supplementation may be necessary, especially for those who have limited sun exposure or live in northern climates.

5. B Vitamins: B vitamins play crucial roles in energy metabolism, nerve function, and red blood cell production. Sources of B vitamins in a gluten-free diet include fortified gluten-free cereals, eggs, dairy products, meat, fish, and leafy greens. However, supplementation may be necessary for some individuals, particularly those with malabsorption issues.

7. **Iron**: Iron deficiency anemia is prevalent among individuals with celiac disease due to intestinal damage that impairs iron absorption. Incorporate iron-rich foods such as lean meats,

poultry, fish, beans, lentils, tofu, spinach, and fortified gluten-free cereals. Iron supplementation may also be recommended in some cases.

8.

7. Omega-3 Fatty Acids: Incorporating sources of omega-3 fatty acids, such as fatty fish (salmon, mackerel, sardines), flaxseeds, chia seeds, and walnuts, can help support heart and brain health. Consider fish oil supplements if dietary intake is insufficient.

8. Probiotics: Individuals with celiac disease or gluten sensitivity may experience imbalances in gut bacteria due to intestinal inflammation. Probiotic supplements or fermented foods like yogurt, kefir, sauerkraut, and kimchi can help restore gut health and support digestion.

9. Consultation with a Registered Dietitian: Since gluten-free diets can be restrictive and may lead to nutritional deficiencies if not properly planned, consulting with a registered dietitian who specializes in gluten-free nutrition is advisable. A dietitian can provide personalized recommendations, meal plans, and guidance on supplementation based on individual needs and preferences.

By incorporating these nutritional considerations and supplements into your gluten-free lifestyle, you can ensure that your dietary choices support optimal health and well-being. Remember to focus on nutrient-dense, whole foods, prioritize variety, and consult with healthcare professionals as needed to address any specific nutritional concerns.

Managing Celiac Disease and Gluten Sensitivity

Managing celiac disease and gluten sensitivity requires more than just avoiding gluten-containing foods; it involves a holistic approach to health and nutrition. Individuals with celiac disease must adhere strictly to a gluten-free diet to prevent damage to the small intestine and alleviate symptoms. Those with gluten sensitivity also benefit from avoiding gluten to prevent discomfort and inflammation. Below are key strategies for managing these conditions and maintaining optimal health on a gluten-free diet:

Understanding Nutritional Needs: When transitioning to a gluten-free diet, it's essential to ensure that nutritional needs are met. Since many gluten-containing grains are fortified with essential nutrients like iron and B vitamins, individuals on a gluten-free diet may be at risk of deficiencies if they don't replace these nutrients with gluten-free alternatives. The "Gluten-Free Food List" book provides guidance on selecting nutrient-rich foods to support overall health and well-being.

Balanced Diet Planning: Following a gluten-free diet doesn't mean sacrificing balanced nutrition. It's important to include a variety of fruits, vegetables, lean proteins, and gluten-free grains in meals to ensure adequate intake of essential nutrients. The book offers meal planning tips and recipes to help individuals create well-rounded, gluten-free meals that meet their nutritional needs.

Choosing Gluten-Free Alternatives: Fortunately, there are many gluten-free alternatives available for commonly consumed gluten-containing foods. From bread and pasta to snacks and desserts, individuals with celiac disease or gluten sensitivity can still enjoy a diverse and satisfying diet. The "Gluten-Free Food List" book provides recommendations for gluten-free products and brands to make shopping easier and more convenient.

Reading Labels: Learning to read food labels is essential for avoiding hidden sources of gluten. Ingredients like modified food starch, malt extract, and hydrolyzed vegetable protein may contain gluten and should be avoided. The book educates readers on how to identify gluten-containing ingredients and choose safe products that are certified gluten-free.

Managing Cross-Contamination: Cross-contamination can occur when gluten-free foods come into contact with gluten-containing foods during preparation, cooking, or serving. Individuals with celiac disease or gluten sensitivity must take precautions to prevent cross-contamination in their kitchens and when dining out. The "Gluten-

Free Food List" book provides practical tips for minimizing the risk of cross-contamination and safely enjoying gluten-free meals.

Monitoring Symptoms: Even with strict adherence to a gluten-free diet, some individuals with celiac disease or gluten sensitivity may continue to experience symptoms due to factors like accidental gluten ingestion or other underlying health conditions. It's essential to monitor symptoms closely and consult with healthcare professionals if symptoms persist or worsen.

Managing celiac disease and gluten sensitivity requires a comprehensive approach that includes strict adherence to a gluten-free diet, nutritional awareness, and proactive measures to prevent cross-contamination. The "Gluten-Free Food List" book serves as a valuable resource for individuals navigating a gluten-free lifestyle, providing practical guidance, and empowering them to make informed choices for their health and well-being.

Gluten-Free and Weight Management

Maintaining a healthy weight while following a gluten-free diet is a common concern for many individuals, especially considering the prevalence of gluten-free processed foods that may be high in sugar, fat, and calories. However, with careful planning and mindful food choices, it is entirely possible to achieve and maintain a healthy weight on a gluten-free diet.

One of the challenges of a gluten-free diet is the tendency to rely on processed gluten-free products, such as bread, pasta, and baked goods, which can be higher in calories and lower in fiber compared to their gluten-containing counterparts. These products often contain refined flours and added sugars to improve texture and taste, but they may lack the essential nutrients found in whole grains.

To manage weight effectively on a gluten-free diet, focus on incorporating nutrient-dense, whole foods into your meals and snacks. Emphasize fresh fruits and vegetables, lean proteins, healthy fats, and gluten-free whole grains like quinoa, brown rice, and buckwheat. These foods provide essential vitamins, minerals, fiber, and protein to support overall health and satiety, helping to prevent overeating and promote weight management.

Another consideration for weight management on a gluten-free diet is portion control. It's easy to overeat on gluten-free snacks and convenience foods, especially if you're not paying attention to portion sizes. Use measuring cups, spoons, and food scales to portion out appropriate serving sizes, and be mindful of your hunger and fullness cues to avoid overeating.

In addition to focusing on whole foods and portion control, regular physical activity is essential for weight management and overall health. Incorporate a combination of cardiovascular exercise, strength training, and flexibility exercises into your routine to support weight loss, improve fitness levels, and reduce the risk of chronic diseases associated with obesity.

Lastly, be mindful of hidden sources of calories, such as sugary beverages, fried foods, and high-calorie snacks. Choose water, herbal tea, or unsweetened beverages instead of sugary sodas and juices, opt for grilled or baked foods instead of fried items, and choose nutrient-dense snacks like fresh fruit, nuts, and yogurt instead of processed snacks.

By focusing on whole foods, portion control, regular physical activity, and mindful eating habits, you can effectively manage your weight on a gluten-free diet while supporting overall health and well-being. Our "Gluten-Free Food List" book provides valuable guidance and resources to help you make informed food choices and achieve your weight management goals while following a gluten-free lifestyle.

Conclusion

In conclusion, embarking on a gluten-free lifestyle can be both empowering and rewarding for individuals managing gluten-related disorders or seeking to improve their overall health. The "Gluten-Free Food List" serves as a valuable resource and companion on this journey, providing comprehensive information, practical tips, and delicious recipes to support individuals in successfully navigating a gluten-free diet.

By understanding the nuances of gluten, identifying safe and hidden sources of gluten, and learning how to make informed food choices, individuals can effectively manage their gluten-related conditions and alleviate symptoms associated with gluten intolerance or celiac disease. The detailed lists of gluten-free foods to enjoy, along with guidance on meal planning and preparation, empower individuals to embrace a diverse and nutritious diet without compromising taste or satisfaction.

Moreover, the "Gluten-Free Food List" emphasizes the importance of gluten-free certification and the significance of choosing products that meet stringent gluten-free standards. By opting for certified gluten-free products and being vigilant about label reading, individuals can minimize the risk of accidental gluten exposure and enjoy peace of mind knowing that their dietary choices align with their health goals.

Furthermore, the book recognizes the challenges and obstacles that may arise when following a gluten-free diet, such as dining out, social gatherings, and traveling. It offers practical tips and strategies for navigating these situations with confidence, ensuring that individuals can maintain their gluten-free lifestyle wherever they go.

Ultimately, the "Gluten-Free Food List" is more than just a compilation of safe foods; it's a comprehensive guide that empowers individuals to take control of their health and well-being through mindful dietary choices. Whether you're newly diagnosed with celiac disease, managing gluten sensitivity, or simply exploring the benefits of a gluten-free lifestyle, this book provides the knowledge, support, and inspiration needed to thrive on your gluten-free journey. As you embark on this path, may you discover newfound vitality, enjoyment, and freedom in embracing a gluten-free way of life.

www.ingramcontent.com/pod-product-compliance
Lightning Source LLC
Chambersburg PA
CBHW050812250726
48653CB00006B/2185